100 Self-Care Ideas for Parents

Freeda Meighan

Contents

Introduction

Being a parent is one of the most wonderful and challenging things you can be in life. Thus, it is important for parents to make time for themselves, so they can remain healthy and happy. Making time to pamper yourself is one of the best things you can do as a parent. It not only keeps your mind healthy but also gives you more energy and focus to take care of the people who depend on you.

Self-care is an important aspect of good parenting. As a parent, it is easy to forget about taking care of yourself while you run around in circles trying to be everything for everyone else. The truth is that if you are not in a position to provide your best self, then it becomes difficult to do your best as a parent. Without self-care, you may find yourself dealing with exhaustion and burnout sooner than you expect. No one is truly one hundred percent selfless, but you need to take care of yourself in order to take care of your family.

Taking time for self-care doesn't mean that you're selfish. It means that you respect yourself enough to take care of your needs and feel good about them. Self-care isn't a self-centered act. In fact, the more you take care of your own needs, the better you can take care of others.

However, self-care can be difficult to fit in, especially if you are a new parent. The majority of new parents don't make time for themselves because they feel too preoccupied with taking care of everyone else. This is the moment when you need to stand up and say: "enough!" You owe it both to yourself and to your family members to take time every day for self-care.

There are many different types of self-care practices. Even looking at pictures or listening to relaxing music may count as self-care. The important thing is that these activities help you relax, relieve stress, and revitalize your mind and body. The first step towards good self-care is being aware of how your mind reacts when you let down your defenses. If you find it difficult to relax, ask yourself why. You may be feeling too tired or burned out from taking care of your family all the time. Practice deep breathing exercises and meditation until you feel more relaxed and centered.

You will find that stress can build up in every aspect of your life, letting go of things that no longer serve you is one good way to let go of some stress. It is significant for parents to find the time to do something for themselves. By making this a priority, you will find that your family is better off too.

When you take the time to care for yourself, you will find that your life is filled with more joy and positive energy. You will feel better about yourself and your role as a parent, making it easier to give your family all the love and care that they need.

Remember that no one can be completely noble and altruistic at all times, therefore self-care is necessary for everyone. If you have young children or other dependents, however, it is especially important to practice self-care on a regular basis. The better job you do taking care of yourself, the more capable you are of taking care of everyone else in your family. When you make time for yourself, you help yourself become a better parent, friend, partner, and individual.

Self-care doesn't have to be complicated or expensive. There are plenty of ways to pamper yourself as a parent that will make you feel invigorated and refreshed. Hopefully, these simple ideas from this short book can help you keep the stress at bay so your body and mind can thrive.

Just because self-care is simple doesn't mean it isn't powerful. You can take care of yourself in a variety of ways, from eating a healthy diet to getting good sleep to giving yourself time for exercise. It sounds obvious, but you will feel better when your body gets what it needs on a daily basis—and you will have more energy and mental clarity in general.

100 Self-Care Ideas for Parents

1. Have a "me time" day.

Spend one day every week doing nothing but what you want. This may be going for a stroll, watching your favorite TV show, or reading that book you've been wanting to read. The remainder of the week is spent doing things for others, such as cooking, doing laundry, aiding with schooling, and so on. Taking care of oneself, on the other hand, does not have to be an all-or-nothing concept.

2. Get a massage.

Allow yourself to enjoy a massage, whether it's a back rub or a foot rub from your partner, or perhaps a great calming massage at the spa. It doesn't have to be on a regular basis, and there are several ways to give yourself this treat.

3. Pamper yourself with a facial.

Getting pampered, whether it's with an aromatherapy facial or a treatment for blackheads and other skin imperfections, can boost your confidence. To get rid of extra dead skin cells, you can also use an exfoliating scrub or face mask. You'll treat yourself, and your skin will look better as a result.

4. Have a warm bath or shower.

For half an hour, forget about everything and simply be in the moment. Add some candles, your favorite music, and anything else that will help you achieve that 'zen' state. The faster you achieve this state of mind, the more likely it is to lift you out of a negative mood or stressful situation.

5. Make time to exercise or work out daily.

Every day is a fantastic chance to be active. There are several benefits to exercising, whether you go to the gym, cycle, or simply walk around the block. A little workout, even if only for ten minutes, can lower stress levels. Working out can also improve your sleep.

6. Visit a friend.

Not everyone is fortunate to have a great number of friends, but even if you just have one friend who is nice to you, spending time with these people may make you feel amazing. So phone someone you like and check if you can drop by.

7. Get out into nature.

You may go for a walk in the woods or along the nearby shore. Getting some fresh air and sunlight often helps to put things into perspective. People frequently overlook how lovely the world is, and there is nothing like it to help us unwind.

8. Plan a night out.

When you need to get away from it all, why not organize a nice meal or movie with your partner? Simply doing something different can help to divert your attention away from your problems for a while. Plus, who can refuse an evening out with their special someone? It's also pleasant to be able to get dressed up after a long day. If you can't find someone to babysit your children, you may do it at home while they sleep on the porch or patio.

9. Spend time with your pets.

Having a pet used to be an expensive responsibility, and people didn't always grasp the idea of adopting one. However, these days, you may not only have animals for free, but they also bring companionship to both children and adults, so why not take advantage? They love us unconditionally, and listening to them purr is thought to be beneficial for your health.

10. Play video or board games.

Letting off some steam with your family and friends is made easy with video games or board games. Not only are they fun, but they can also help to alleviate stress. Video games, in particular, have proven to be an effective way of reducing anxiety. Plus, you're sure to enjoy lots of laughter and distraction from whatever it was that had you feeling overwhelmed.

11. Create a family day out.

Why not plan a weekly outing with the whole family? Taking some time to get away from work and enjoy each others' company could be something as simple as having a picnic on the beach or lunch at the park. This allows you to cultivate strong relationships outside of your working hours, all while strengthening bonds within your family.

12. Go for a walk.

The '10,000 steps a day' goal is one that many people enjoy striving for. However, it's not necessary to hit the full 10K if you don't want to. Self-care isn't about pushing yourself into activities you dislike — something as straightforward as strolling around your neighborhood or local park can be just as beneficial. The most important thing is that any exercise gets those feet moving. After all, movement equals health and happiness.

13. Dance it out.

Don't let the fear of having "two left feet" stop you from getting on the dance floor with your partner. Whether it's in the living room, bedroom, kitchen, or any other space that strikes your fancy — have fun by playing something upbeat and engaging to really get into the groove. Put on a classic club tune, play some music you both love, or even dust off that disco record that has been collecting dust for years. Do whatever gets those two left feet moving.

14. Sing along to your favorite song.

Unleash your inner voice and share the joy of singing. Let whatever tune makes you happy and be part of a chorus that only you can lead. Regardless if it's an upbeat or heartfelt melody, just find what brings out a smile within and sing to the world.

15. Put your feet up.

After a hectic day, you likely find solace in "putting your feet up" on the couch. This age-old expression is commonly associated with comfort and relaxation precisely because it offers many physical benefits. Elevating your legs at a 90-degree angle against a surface helps restore blood flow to your heart while promoting lymphatic fluid circulation throughout the body, allowing it to truly recover and recharge. So next time, after an arduous day, don't forget to put those feet up for some much-deserved rest and recuperation.

16. Find a new hobby.

While it's not always easy, activities like hobbies can help to lift your spirits while simultaneously providing a distraction from negative thoughts. So why not find something you have an aptitude for and make sure that when engaging in it, you don't become fixated on all of the things you haven't mastered yet? A successful hobby can be incredibly beneficial.

17. Light aromatherapy candles.

After a hectic day and your energy depleted, all you want is for the night to come quickly so that you can hit the sack. However, lighting some candles at this point will give you enough time to relax before retiring for the evening.

18. Get a manicure and pedicure.

Experience the ultimate relaxation with a luxurious manicure and pedicure. You don't need to visit the salon — you can achieve professional results right in your own home using polish, files, and more. Plus, giving yourself a flawless at-home manicure is surprisingly easy.

19. Read an inspiring book.

Take some time to nourish your soul by immersing yourself in a book that will fill you with optimism and motivation. Choose something that speaks to you, something which knows how to move the heart as well as enlighten the mind. There is no better way than surrendering yourself wholeheartedly into an inspirational page-turner.

20. Practice Yoga.

Unwind and find inner peace with yoga. Dozens of studios offer different types of practice, so take some time to choose one that resonates with you. Or seek counsel from your doctor on which classes would suit you best.

21. Listen to relaxing music.

The soul can be calmed by contemplative, deep music. You may need something to divert your attention from troubling thoughts when it seems as though your life is imploding around you. You could feel happier if you listen to upbeat music. After a hard day, listening to music is a wonderful way to unwind, and its therapeutic benefits are well-recognized.

22. Listen to audiobooks.

When performing tasks like cleaning the dishes or folding clothes, audiobooks are a terrific alternative to music to listen to. Even if it seems a little ridiculous at first, it doesn't take long until you become used to having someone tell you an amazing story while you do something else, especially if that person is an exceptional narrator.

23. Read uplifting articles from credible news sources online.

Read the stories of people who are making positive changes in their communities to improve the environment. These sites can both entertain and offer expert advice that will help you on those bad days when nothing seems right.

24. Practice meditation.

Meditation lowers blood pressure and heart rates, reducing stress-related symptoms such as anxiety. It also reduces levels of cortisol (a hormone that keeps people alert). Guided meditations can be especially soothing, but you could also try taking a class to get some guidance in learning how to do it properly.

25. Buy yourself some flowers.

Your day may be made better by beautiful flowers, especially if you're experiencing a bad day. You may get them from a grocery shop or a florist. Make time to relax with a bouquet at home. Even better, these lovely flowers can inspire you to spend more time on yourself when you have some "me-time."

26. Cook a special dish for your family.

Perhaps you have a favorite dish that brings back memories of your childhood. Cook it, or perhaps utilize a traditional family recipe that your grandma used to prepare for you. Give yourself and others around you the gift of something good and nutritious.

27. Bake something delicious with your kids.

You will be teaching positive habits to them by sharing your love for cooking, even if they are too little to partake. You are sure to enjoy preparing a variety of family-friendly cakes and pastries together.

28. Go on a salon/spa date with your partner.

Getting your hair done, getting a hot stone massage, or experiencing an aromatherapy steam room can definitely help improve your attitude and spirits. Furthermore, spending time with your partner makes you feel closer to him.

29. Clean the house together.

If your home has become cluttered, it may be a terrific opportunity for your family to spend time together while helping each other achieve something. Cleaning the house can also be a lot of fun for children. Making it a competition by offering the kids tiny rewards for "cleaning" the house is a good idea.

30. Watch your favorite TV show together as a family.

Simply watch your favorite TV show with your partner and children and relinquish all parental obligations for the time being. Having the same sentiments as each other might bring you closer together. This activity provides that sense of connectedness. Likewise, this is a wonderful way to bond as a couple or as a family.

31. Go to your favorite restaurant.

If you don't dine out much, you might want to sometimes indulge in delicious meals at your favorite restaurant. You can spend your "me time" alone, or perhaps it would be wise to organize a family get-together by going to that restaurant where the server usually brings you extra bread and remembers your name. It will give you the confidence boost you need.

32. Watch your favorite movies.

This one is perfect for self-care as well. It is amazing to see a movie with a special someone and cry or laugh along at the end of the film. Plan a weekend movie marathon if you want to see movies you like or haven't watched before.

33. Learn knitting or sewing.

For all kinds of crafts, there are many superb YouTube videos available. Try knitting or sewing something for your partner if you feel comfortable doing so. This is not only a pleasant present, but the act of making something also makes you feel closer to one another.

34. Learn how to play an instrument.

Something about playing an instrument is simply so amazing and delightful. You can find time to practice and play while also working to hone your abilities. When you're feeling low, try to surround yourself with as much music as you can.

35. Grow plants even in small spaces.

Try growing plants if you have a space, even a little cup on your windowsill. While taking care of it, you have something lovely to gaze at. Your feelings are lifted as you watch it flourish because you feel more connected to nature.

36. Diffuse essential oils around the house.

Essential oils are excellent for easing tension and anxiety in people. Place some of them in a diffuser, or even in bowls throughout your home, or dab some of it on your wrists.

37. Listen to a podcast.

Listening to podcasts is a terrific way to learn about people's experiences in many professions, gain knowledge from experts, or simply laugh along with their jokes. Through discussions on personal interests or issues that can arise at work, podcast topics can also provide you with a chance to improve your relationship with your partner.

38. Talk about fun memories with your kids.

Consider sharing a happy memory with your kids if you're going through a difficult time. You can share your own fond recollections of your childhood and the activities you enjoyed, or you can elicit their most treasured childhood memories. This will not only be an enjoyable way to interact with them, but it will also jog your memory of happy moments that may come in handy for them as they go through their own challenging times.

39. Go camping.

Given that you just need to pack the bare minimum, including food and water, it's not only exciting and adventurous but also less expensive. A tent and sleeping bag should be brought along. You'll also get the chance to reconnect with nature, which is something you may not do frequently.

40. Go boating/sailing.

The steady, consistent hum of an engine or the sound of the water can provide great relaxation. It's also not as pricey as you may think. See what kinds of boats are available for hire by contacting your local boat club, which is generally listed online.

41. Learn to surf together.

Everyone may go at their own pace when surfing, so you can enjoy it with your children. No prior swimming experience is necessary for beginner lessons, which are conducted in shallow water with other newbies. The entire family will have a fantastic time engaging in this activity since everyone will get to watch one another surf.

42. Drive somewhere you've never been before.

You could always accomplish this on the weekend. Simply choose a direction and begin driving. Locate a route with amazing views, then look for a new restaurant for lunch or dinner.

43. Get yourself a treat at the grocery store.

Purchase a box of your favorite granola bar or cereal and keep it on hand whenever you feel like something quick to eat. A little treat you may have been meaning to try may be purchased here as well, giving you yet another thing to look forward to.

44. Plan art activities for the family.

You may get puzzle-making kits or print out some doodle art. Perhaps you could snap some pictures of your kids having fun, frame them, and place them on the wall.

45. Paint the walls.

Your house will feel much different after receiving a great coat or two of paint. It could make you feel rejuvenated and full of optimism. Although this pastime might not be for everyone, if you're having a rough day, go purchase some paint and repaint some walls. To feel better in your home environment, get rid of the old hue and develop something fresh.

46. Get some new clothing.

Consider buying some new outfits or shoes to celebrate if you're feeling down and your wardrobe is in horrible shape. It might be hard to find something you love, but it's great to treat yourself to new items. Doing things for yourself is perfectly fine; don't feel bad.

47. Make happy picture collages.

With your camera or smartphone, you may create collages out of your family pictures. Make them seem fancier by adding embellishments or frills. Create one for your family when you're depressed so that you don't forget to find something to be joyful about every day, even if it's only a small thing.

48. Go to the park and feed the ducks.

This may be one of your favorite things to do when the weather is nice. Sit by the lake with some bread you picked up from the grocery store or nearby bakery while you see the numerous joyful birds flying around in search of food.

49. Go to a museum you've never been to.

Every city has a ton of them, and some of them are even free. Simply explore everything for a few hours. Don't worry about what other people may think - simply enjoy the work. Take some photographs, then tell someone else about your discovery.

50. Go hiking.

Hiking is a great way for the family to receive lots of fresh air, sunshine, and exercise if there is a nearby spot. Your children can pick their favorite clothing if you decide where you're going in advance so they'll be comfortable on the trek. When the kids are at school, you may also do this by yourself. Just make sure that it is safe for solo hikers.

51. Find a place that serves foreign cuisines.

Your family will love the selection of food, and you could possibly find some tasty bargains on unique dishes to try. Ask your loved ones what they think after tasting something new! This can be a great opportunity for everyone to bond together as well.

52. Listen to live music with friends.

Why not lift yourself out of a low mood with the perfect combination — friends, food, and music? What could be better than tuning into tunes that you love while in good company, surrounded by individuals who have similar interests to your own? Rather than just streaming from Spotify or Apple Music, why not treat yourself to an even more immersive experience and find an area for some real-life bands instead?

53. Find a new scenic place to take pictures.

Have you recently experienced the beauty of a sunrise or sunset? Or marveled at an intriguing tree or cloud-covered mountain range? Take a stroll and discover where your camera can capture some breathtaking views.

54. Go see a comedy show and improv performances.

Make sure to stop in at a nearby comedy club or improv theater. With so many of these venues scattered across the country, you're certain to find one (or several) close by. Check out an open mic night — you'll get away from home for a bit, show your support for local talent, and enjoy plenty of hearty laughter.

55. Find an animal shelter near you.

Locate an animal shelter nearby and visit it with your family members. Make a difference by adopting, volunteering at the facility, or even supplying food. An ideal opportunity to show your children how to take care of animals awaits you.

56. Go to a self-help or psychology bookstore.

Why not explore the selection of books that capture your attention, even if they are just the newest bestsellers? If possible and allowed, grab a book or two along with a cup of coffee and settle into an inviting couch or chair for some free reading pleasure.

57. Watch some awesome TED Talks.

Are you searching for something that can be truly inspiring, educational, and informative? Find a video about your passion- whatever it is in life that ignites the spark within you but has been left untapped due to all of life's obligations. By discovering this, you will come to understand yourself better and feel empowered as ever before.

58. Donate blood.

Contributing blood offers immense physical and mental advantages. Not only do you acquire a gratis snack, but you also get the rewarding feeling of having saved someone's life. Furthermore, the idle time between donations makes for an ideal opportunity to have some personal time!

59. Organize a cook-off with your partner.

For an enjoyable evening, invite your friends over and create teams to whip up a delicious dish. Afterward, you can have the winners judged by either all of the participants or just let the children decide who made the best presentation or most creative meal. Get ready for some intense competition.

60. Find some place like a farmer's market or flea market to walk around.

Forget the mundane items you can buy in a big box store. When it comes to finding special and unique things, often at bargain prices, handmade items are your best bet. Keep an eye out for sales on both practical replacements you need as well as some exquisite gadgets and trinkets that will make even better treats for yourself.

61. Plan a staycation at the hotel nearby.

You deserve to relax because you worked hard all week. With your family, stay at a hotel. Watch a movie, get room service for dinner, go swimming in the pool or hot tub — do whatever appeals to you. Just allow yourself to take it easy for a few days.

62. Watch foreign drama shows.

These are fantastic mood boosters. You should look online to see what amazing shows are now airing. These international programs will have you swooning, despite how cheesy it sounds. These are also excellent ways to learn about the cultures and the way of life of other countries.

63. Learn a foreign language with the family.

This is a terrific way to stimulate your brain while learning something new. Actual foreign languages like Spanish or French can be included in this. Learn how to use endearing language and address your lover in it. This activity will undoubtedly be a hit with kids. While challenging, doing this may be enjoyable.

64. Purchase a new watch as a gift to one another.

Consider it a gift on your anniversary. If both of you enjoy watches or other timepieces, this is a terrific way to relax with your sweetheart.

65. Take an online fitness class.

Even while you can always find one for free on YouTube or other websites, some well-known fitness instructors also have websites where you may pay to take one. It is an ideal way to get good exercise and gives you something to look forward to each day.

66. Make your own fruit smoothies.

Online recipe resources are abundant. It's a terrific way to get your recommended daily intake of fruits, veggies, and other nutritious foods. Plus, it's more convenient than buying them pre-made.

67. Recycle or find new uses for old things.

This is a wonderful approach to doing a task when you're short on time. You may reuse clothing by hanging it up or store plastic bags in your drawers to make them more functional. It won't take long for you to discover dozens of household recycling options. It's beneficial on two levels: it saves you money by preventing you from purchasing things brand-new and it lessens waste by keeping stuff out of landfills.

68. Go stargazing.

It is an amazing way to get out of the house at night and disconnect from devices. It's a fact that most individuals spend their whole workday engrossed in their phones or computer displays. Therefore, stargazing is beneficial for the soul.

69. Enroll in a pottery class.

If you want to do something both creative and hands-on, but don't find traditional arts appealing, why not try a pottery class? This activity is an excellent way to improve your hand strength, wrist mobility, and arm muscles. Not only that, but it also offers the opportunity for knowledge acquisition in this field — plus, you can make lovely mementos for those dear to you.

70. Take silly selfies.

Enhance your confidence and showcase your unique sense of style by taking a selfie in something fashionable. Not only will it make you happy for the rest of the day, but it'll also serve as an inspirational reminder that you are in control of your life.

71. Start a blog.

Now is the perfect opportunity to do something you've always wanted to do. You will have the chance to be creative and express all of your feelings as a parent by starting a blog. It's likely that many others share your sentiments, and discovering them online may make life more fun. So don't worry if no one reads it.

72. Read comic books with your kids.

You may have read superhero comics and classic fairy tales as a child, but have you ever read them as a parent? Use this instructive platform to present them to your children. It's a terrific method for parents to unwind and take a quick break by reading comic books. Read aloud to your child in turns, and then talk about what is occurring in the story. Some of these classics are available for borrowing at your local library, or you can purchase them at discount prices from used bookstores or online stores like Amazon.

73. Drink warm milk before bedtime.

The quality of sleep can be improved by having a warm drink before bed. If you want to improve digestion and strengthen your immunity, incorporate a glass of warm milk into your diet.

74. Take some online courses related to your hobbies.

Consider taking a photography class, a cooking course, a baking class, or a history class on a period that interests you. You could discover that learning something new online or through Massive Open Online Courses (MOOCs) is more economical and enjoyable than at your nearby institution.

75. Play gentle wrestling with your kid.

Like what you see on TV, you probably pictured a strong man tossing another strong man. This time, it is not intended to be done that way. Try playing "wrestle" in the house with your toddler; roll around on the floor with them and take short breaks to tickle their backs or tummies. Both of you will enjoy this, and it can teach them how to manage their body.

76. Do something spontaneous.

When was the last time you traveled or engaged in an activity without first making a plan? Try doing something a bit different from what you typically do, whether it's going on an unplanned date or just going to an amusement park on a whim.

77. Send sweet messages to your spouse.

While you're focused on your job, it's simple to overlook the people you care about. A charming, amicable, and motivating note to your partner could make them grin. To express how much you value all your spouse does for you and your family, send your spouse a quick text or email to let them know you're thinking of them.

78. Drink wine together

A lovely moment that may potentially strengthen your relationship is sharing a great bottle of wine over dinner. A long-term happy marriage is more likely for couples who love simple things together.

79. Make your hygiene routine more relaxing.

Research has revealed that warm showers and scented soaps can make people feel a sense of calm. Take the opportunity to give yourself some much-needed TLC each day by setting aside time for hygiene practices like taking baths or showers. If you prefer baths over showers, enjoy one after your little ones have gone to sleep in the evening. It not only allows you to relax but also gives your body an opportunity to close out stress before bedtime. Make sure it's enjoyable too. Light up your favorite fragrant candles, play calming music, and use a loofah mitt for extra indulgence.

80. Mix up your routine.

Try switching things up and doing something different if you find yourself in the same spot every day. You might be surprised by how much it could help improve your mood.

81. Research and share interesting facts.

Exploring and learning new things can be a fun way to connect with your friends and family. Plus, it's self-care. Not only does sharing something you're passionate about bring joy to those around you, but everyone loves discovering something fresh.

82. Find volunteer work.

Are you passionate about a certain cause or topic? If so, there are likely plenty of charitable organizations out there in search of volunteers like you. Even if your ultimate mission is not to save the world overnight, rendering aid and assistance to others can elevate both their lives as well as yours.

83. Travel abroad with the family.

There is no better way to spend quality time with your family than traveling together. Exploring the world is an incredible experience and a remarkable opportunity for all members of the family. Uniting in escapades abroad or day trips out of town provides moments that last forever — from bonding and seeing new places, to making memories. These are invaluable gifts you can give each other by traveling as a family.

84. Go skydiving, bungee jumping, or snowboarding.

Ready to make your wildest dreams come true? Taking action in this area of your life could be one of the most rewarding experiences you can have. So what are you waiting for? Start taking steps towards achieving something remarkable today.

85. Call a friend that you haven't talked to in a while.

Feeling low? Don't let yourself drift away from the people who care about you. Instead, be proactive and reach out to them! Call, text, or email - whatever works for you. Don't wait around expecting someone else to make that first move. Take the initiative and stay connected with your loved ones.

86. Stop watching the news.

For the time being, at least. Try to refrain from reading or viewing news that may bring you a negative vibe. We are all aware of how stressful and distressing it is to listen to or be subjected to excessive quantities of fear-mongering. You don't need to add unneeded negativity to your stress.

87. Unplug from technology that stresses you out.

At least an hour before going to sleep, unplug any gadgets. After attempting to get some sleep, wait three hours before checking your phone or computer. When you wake up in the morning, avoid checking Facebook, Twitter, or any other social networking site. Seeing crazy news stories will make you anxious, especially when your brain is already under stress.

88. Create your own self-care package.

Pick things that will make you feel better during challenging times. These objects should be placed in a compact box, which should be kept wherever it is constantly accessible and visible. Candles, confections, little bottles of essential oils, acupressure bands, and headphones for listening to music are a few examples of self-care items.

89. Create a "do not disturb" zone.

Make sure this space is uncluttered and unobstructed, whether it is at home or at work. It may be a moment when there are no interruptions, including phone calls. Do all in your power to give yourself the time and space to take care of yourself.

90. Identify what specifically brings you down.

For instance, if you care about someone and haven't heard from them in a while, call them or arrange a get-together.

91. Write down your thoughts and emotions in a journal.

Keeping a journal has been clinically shown to be an invaluable tool for emotional well-being. With writing, you can confront difficult feelings and explore them with self-compassion. By putting the words on paper, it not only allows you to look at your thoughts more closely but also serves as an act of self-love that seeks understanding rather than judgment.

92. Reread any inspiring quotes you find comforting.

It's beneficial to have sources of encouragement and mantras that you can revisit when your emotions take a turn. One optimistic concept often leads to the next, providing a spark for motivation.

93. Attend a worship service.

Embracing prayer and gratitude can be a powerful source of comfort when you feel overwhelmed. Worshiping is an incredible way to navigate the struggles that arise daily. Whether it's close to home or far away, uplifting words from spiritual teachings will replenish your spirit and lift your burdens.

94. Make it a point to hug your partner everyday.

If you fail to keep your relationship alive, then it has the potential of gradually deteriorating without alerting you. Hugs have a remarkable effect on our well-being - they can ease stress hormones, strengthen immunity, and help us bond with someone special.

95. Update your style.

From something small like wearing a new pair of earrings to anything daring such as splurging on hair extensions or getting a trendy tattoo, it's always rewarding when you look and feel more your style. You don't need to make drastic changes all at once; however, taking the initiative to better yourself will undoubtedly provide immense comfort and joy. Make sure that whatever you decide on is done with pride since you deserve only the best.

96. Go on a retreat for the day.

Everyone needs a break from the hustle and bustle of everyday life, so why not take some time out for an overnight retreat with your partner or close friends? Whether you're looking to disconnect in solitude or simply enjoy quality time together, retreating is sure to provide both! Not only will it offer peace and tranquility, but it will also allow important relationships to be nurtured.

97. Create your own support network.

Finding solidarity with others in a similar situation as you have can generate incredible advantages. Reach out to your family, friends, and even professional counselors. Think outside the box by joining online forums where people are experiencing comparable thoughts or feelings as yourself. Not only will connecting on this level create an understanding of mutual support, but you may also gain insight into managing stress and anxieties from their perspectives.

98. Get plenty of sleep.

Sleep is an important part of recovery and performance, yet many days can be a challenge when you're tired. Instead of forcing yourself to stay awake, try getting 6-8 hours of sleep. There's nothing quite like the sensation you get when your body finally relaxes as soon as your head hits the pillow.

99. Make a list of all your accomplishments.

Reflect on the events, successes, and achievements that bring you pride in your life. It's healthy to take a moment to appreciate what you've accomplished — big or small. Put pen to paper and list out each accomplishment for yourself. Feel good about everything on your list.

100. Write a bucket list.

Have you ever heard of a 'bucket list'? It's essentially an accumulation of all the activities, goals, and life experiences that you want to experience before passing away. You can make one for today, next month, or even your entire lifetime. Furthermore, it is possible to collaborate with your partner on what both of you want to accomplish together. Use this as the perfect opportunity to start chasing after those dreams which are dear to your heart.

Conclusion

Parenting can be a whirlwind of activity, leaving precious little time to take care of yourself. But it's essential that you do! When we include our own needs in the list of priorities and ensure they are met, parenting becomes far less stressful — plus all that relaxation translates into more energy for loving interaction with your children. Self-care is not just important; it makes your family life better overall so you're able to prioritize quality moments with them and make parenting easier than ever before.

Self-care is a vital habit for any parent to have as it provides them with the opportunity to recognize their best self, and ultimately share this version of themselves with their family. Despite how physically and mentally exhausting being a parent can be, studies confirm that caring for oneself while also looking after your children and working is one of life's most difficult responsibilities. Appreciating moments of true self-care allows parents to feel more fulfilled in all aspects of parenting.

It is vital to prioritize self-care in order to maintain physical and mental health, as well as your connection with the world around you. To start, focus on a few simple elements like getting plenty of restful sleep each night and doing something that makes you feel good daily. If there's an issue weighing down on your mind, make sure to address it directly before it snowballs into bigger issues. Self-care can be an invaluable asset if applied correctly.

Investing in your own well-being, and finding moments to do the things that invigorate you, will blossom into great habits. By taking small steps first and ensuring they are achievable goals, it is possible to attain significant outcomes over time.

I hope this book has gifted you with creative ways to add self-care into your hectic lifestyle as a parent. Most importantly, I wish for it to remind you of the immense value in yourself and how important it is that you practice taking care of yourself too!

Leaving a Review

As an independent author with limited marketing resources, reviews for my books are essential in order to survive as an indie writer. New works of literature get published daily, so there's no guarantee that any given work will be successful.

Your review can help authors like me grow and share their knowledge with more people. If you enjoyed this book, I would really appreciate your honest feedback. You can leave a voluntary review by going to this book's page on Amazon, and clicking "Write A Review."

Leaving an honest review can also help other people find this book easily on Amazon and benefit from it as well. Your feedback is important to me so I can find out what you like and don't, which in turn helps me make better decisions about my writing style.

Thank you,

Freeda

More Books to Consider

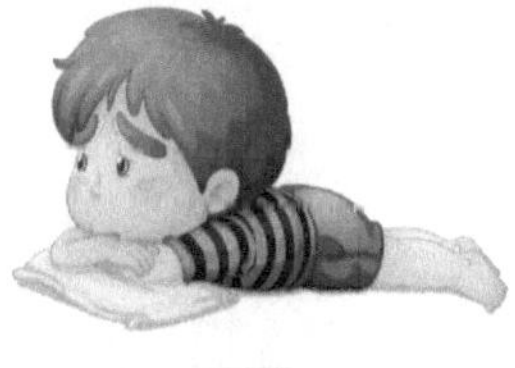

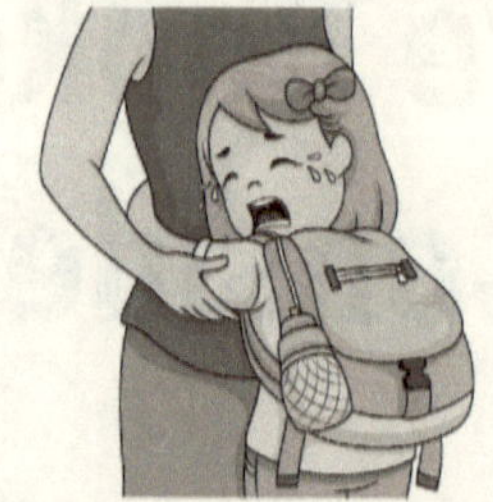
THE EMPATHIC PARENT'S GUIDE TO
RAISING AN
ANXIOUS CHILD
How to Help Your Kids Overcome Shyness,
Worry, Separation and Social Anxiety
FREEDA MEIGHAN

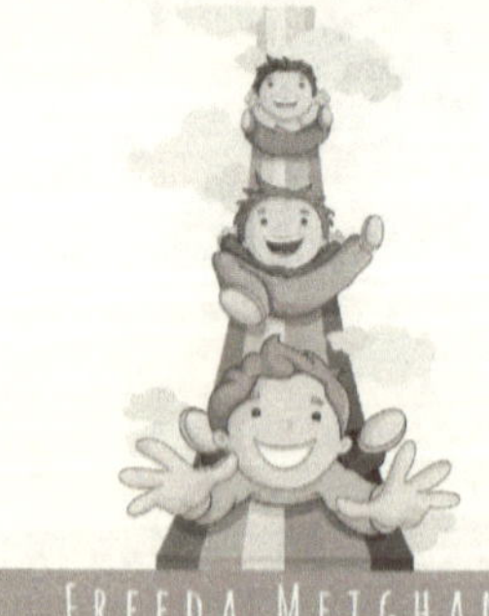
THE EMPATHIC PARENT'S GUIDE TO
RAISING
HAPPY HUMANS
Help Your Children Gain the Virtues
They Need to Live a Good Life
FREEDA MEIGHAN

***

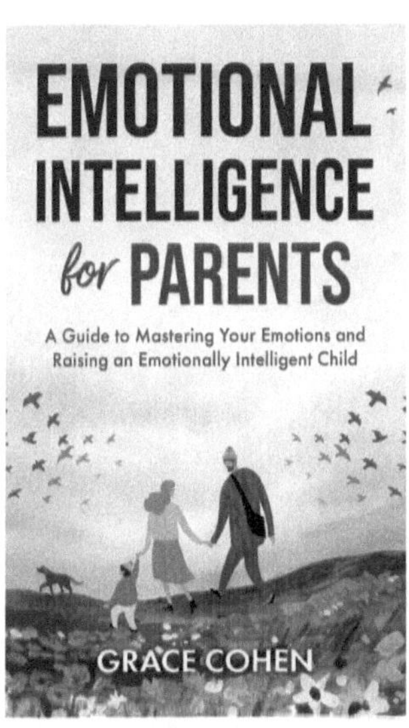

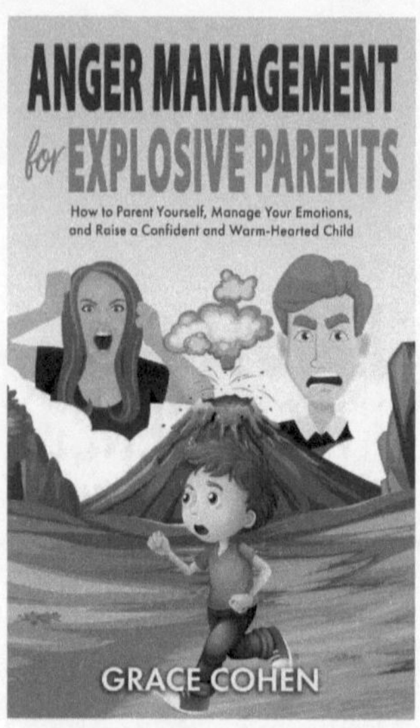
ANGER MANAGEMENT
for EXPLOSIVE PARENTS
How to Parent Yourself, Manage Your Emotions,
and Raise a Confident and Warm-Hearted Child
GRACE COHEN

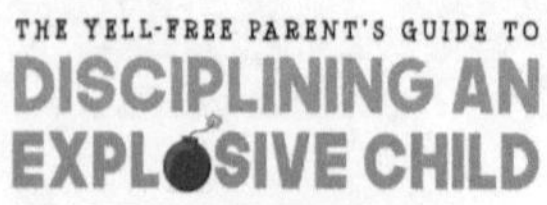
THE YELL-FREE PARENT'S GUIDE TO
DISCIPLINING AN
EXPLOSIVE CHILD
No-Drama Strategies I Discovered to
Discipline My Easily Frustrated Child

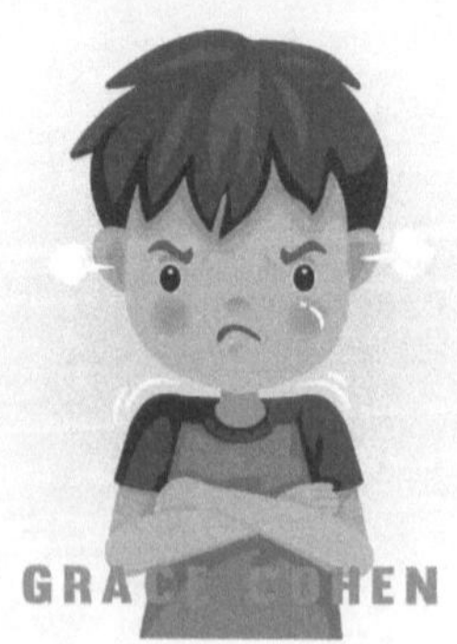
GRACE COHEN

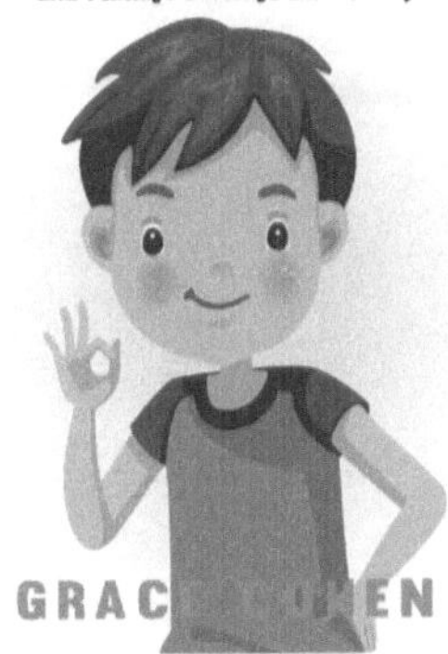
THE YELL-FREE PARENT'S GUIDE TO
RAISING AN
EMPATHIC CHILD
How to Help Your Child Self-Regulate
and Manage Feelings Effectively
GRACE GREEN

About Author

Freeda is a bestselling author who has written multiple books on parenting and family life. She knows that raising children can be tough, but it's also one of the most rewarding experiences any parent can ever have. She has devoted her life to understanding the psychology behind good parenting and shares what she's learned with others through her books, blogs, and newsletters.

She is also a mother of a highly sensitive child. Freeda shares her story not just to help other parents learn how to raise a highly sensitive child but also to impart lessons on what helped her get through the challenges and live a happy life for both herself and her daughter.

After years of navigating the parenting journey herself, Freeda knows that sharing her life experiences with others could help them on their own parenting journeys. She has helped countless mothers, fathers, grandparents, babysitters, and teachers in making their lives easier by providing sound advice from her extensive experience with children's behavior patterns over the years.

In her free time, she goes to her Yoga and Pilates classes. She also loves baking, especially when requested by her children. Their favorite is her bunch of chewy white chocolate macadamia cookies.

Check out Freeda's profile on Amazon: https://www.amazon.com/author/freedameighan